CW00401564

EMERALD GUIDES

A
GUIDE
TO
ALTERNATIVE HEALTH AND
ALTERNATIVE REMEDIES

JENNY HALBERT

Emerald Publishing
www.emeraldpublishing.co.uk

Emerald Guides
Brighton BN2 4EG

ISBN 1847160 52 2
ISBN 13: 9781847160522

Printed by Biddles Ltd Kings Lynn Norfolk
Cover design by Straightforward Graphics

CONTENTS

Introduction

13. Reflexology

14. Relax

15. Think healthy

Useful addresses

Introduction

Many health experts agree that once the body is cleansed, nourished and balanced, it has the ability to heal and recover from disease as well as maintain health and long life. Studies tell us that old age doesn't cause illness. Not everybody who gets old gets sick. By design we're healthy. So how do we lose it? High stress living, processed foods, pollution, and too little exercise all take their toll on our bodies natural vitality. But we can restore our health and increase our vitality through the natural healing arts. These have been with us down through the ages and can be very powerful in engaging and supporting our body's own forces for health and vitality. Our bodies have a strong, innate knowing that works, often miraculously, to achieve a state of balance.

This book serves as an introduction to the various elements which form an alternative to traditional medical remedies as we know them. The book covers remedies in the form of herbal and homeopathic, as well as flower remedies and also covers the essential properties of various types of food. In addition, areas such as aromatherapy, homeopathy and osteopathy are covered. Overall, the book attempts to take a well-balanced look at the area of alternative health, opening up the readers mind to the various possibilities.

Most of us would agree that there are miracles in nature, but how many of us have a sense of wonder for the amazing creatures that we are? Look at your hands. Nothing that man has created excels the human hand in dexterity. And of the 5 billion people in the world, no two fingerprints are the same. If all of our muscles pulled together in one direction, we could lift as much as 25 tons. Not only that, we have a brain that would require a landmass the size of the state of Texas to recreate its full function. You're special. You deserve to be healthy. So read on!

1

ACUPUNCTURE

Acupuncture

Acupuncture is a Chinese treatment which dates back some 2000 years. It involves the use of needles, which are inserted into the skin. In Chinese medicine, the body is thought to possess a network of invisible pathways called meridians, through which a life energy flows. This life energy is known as 'qi' and it comprises two components called yin and yang. The forces of yin and yang are in balance in a healthy person, which allows the qi to flow freely through the meridians, each of which is associated with the different organs. Yin meridians run from the toes or fingertips upwards, yang meridians run from the head to the fingertips or toes. Acupuncturists work with the meridian lines of the body, inserting fine needles to restore the balance of energy in the body by freeing or unblocking the vital energy points.

Acupuncture has often been used for pain relief. However, it can be used to treat various conditions and is particularly useful where inflammation is causing ill-health. Back-pain, arthritis, migraine, menstrual problems, joint pains, high blood pressure, insomnia and cystitis respond well to the treatment. It can be used for pain relief in childbirth and is also widely believed to alleviate emotional problems such as anxiety, stress, depression as well as respiratory ailments and digestive disorders. It is increasingly being incorporated into drug detoxification programs.

One explanation of the way acupuncture works is that a nerve impulse is fired off to the spinal cord from the needle insertion. This has the effect of releasing the body's own natural painkiller, endorphins. Another is the 'gate' theory of pain, where pain impulses are believed to be controlled by a gate along the pathways of the nervous system. Acupuncture is believed to stimulate certain nerve fibers which close the gate and shut off the pain. Acupuncture is also thought to release substances in the brain which induce feelings of drowsiness and relaxation. This has a positive effect on the body's hormones and on the limbic centre in the brain, an area which controls mood and behaviour, and is believed to be concerned with addiction.

After diagnosis, the acupuncturist will place the needles in certain points along selected meridians, the most commonly used points being along the limbs, below the knees and between the elbows and the fingers. The needles are normally made from stainless steel and are almost as fine as hair. There is little or no pain on insertion. Needles are usually inserted to a depth of a centimetre, but depending on the part of the body, insertion can vary from one millimetre to several centimeters. The needles may be left in for up to twenty minutes.

The British Medical Acupuncture Society (BMAS) was formed in 1980 as an association of medical practitioners interested in acupuncture. There are now 1500 members who use acupuncture in hospital or general practice. The BMAS is a registered charity established to stimulate and promote the use and scientific understanding of acupuncture for the benefit of the public.

2

THE ALEXANDER TECHNIQUE

The demands of contemporary life can so occupy our thoughts that we forget about the most important consideration: ourselves. The Alexander Technique encourages correct posture and proper use of our bodies in everyday life. Since all activities from walking, sitting and reading to talking involve the use of many muscles, there is a lot of potential for us to lapse into postural bad habits. These cause excess tension in the muscles, which in turn results in aches and pains and less efficient breathing, circulation and digestion.

The Alexander technique is considered not so much a therapy as effective use of the whole body in everyday activities. Usually it involves a series of lessons in which awareness of the body and posture is enhanced. It confronts the causes of many cases of back pain, neck and shoulder tension, breathing disorders, stress related illnesses and general fatigue where incorrect poise is a contributory factor. Most commonly the Alexander Technique is used for back pain, migraine or joint conditions such as arthritis. Whiplash, repetitive strain injury, stress related conditions and depression can also benefit from it.

15

This treatment was invented by an Austrian actor, F. M. Alexander. He had respiratory problems, and this combined with the stress of his profession began to affect his voice badly and threaten his career, so he devised a specific technique to relax his muscles and cure his failing voice.

By adopting the Alexander technique you will find breathing and speaking become easier, and movement becomes freer, lighter and more enjoyable. The Alexander technique is widely used to improve performance in sports, music and drama. Several music colleges offer Alexander lessons because it helps breathing, pre-performance nerves and releases tension from the muscles around the vocal cords. The technique has been part of a 2 million pound programme funded by the British Performing Arts Medicine Trust to combat stage fright.

3

AROMATHERAPY

Aromatherapy combines pure essences from aromatic plants with the magic of touch. Essential oils have been prized for their health giving qualities for thousands of years, and these oils stimulate the sense of smell which in turn affects the area of the brain thought to control instinctive behaviour, strong emotions and mood control

The essential oils have a complex chemical structure which the body activates by absorbing it through the skin into the bloodstream. The oils are usually massaged into the body, and this helps to release stress in the muscles and promote a feeling of relaxation and well-being. Through correct massage, all functions of the organs of the body - skin, muscles, nerves, glands and so on, are stimulated, and as a result of the increased circulation of the blood and lymph, the clearing away of body waste is more efficient. Body massage movements can range from soft, light, rhythmical stroking movements whose purpose is to relax the muscles and nerves, to heavy pounding and kneading designed to break down fatty areas.

The word massage originates from a Greek word meaning to knead, and it is one of the oldest forms of treatment for ailments. Hippocrates (460-380BC) described treatment for a dislocated shoulder as follows.. "it is necessary to rub the shoulder gently and smoothly with soft hands. The physician must be experienced in many things, but assuredly also in rubbing."

Essential oils are extracted from the flowers, leaves, fruit, seeds and bark of plants by steam distillation. At present there are 400 different plant essences, each with different characteristics and healing properties. These potent, volatile essences are nature's gift to mind, body, and spirit.

The link between emotions and the release of chemicals in the body is well known. Essential oils can evoke imagery; sometimes the smell of a certain aroma can instantly bring back memories of childhood. Some scents can make us feel relaxed while others can make us feel energized and alive - such is the power of aroma. For centuries it has been common knowledge that scents produce mental and physical responses. Due to its impact on the limbic system, aromatherapy can stimulate the release of beneficial chemicals and hormones in the body. Minute molecules of essential oils are carried in the bloodstream and affect different organs.

Aromatherapy has a wide range of uses. Digestive problems, skin conditions, muscular aches, premenstrual tension and menopausal problems all respond well to the treatment. Because it encourages relaxation, aromatherapy is good for all stress related conditions and the aim of the therapy is to support the body in its fight against disease.

The distillation of essential oils began in the Middle East, and the knowledge of how these oils can be used for healing was thought to have been introduced into Europe by the Romans. In Britain, essential oils were popular in the eighteen century but their use dwindled in the nineteenth century due to the rise of orthodox medicine. Aromatherapy was revived in Britain by Robert Tisserand in 1969, and it is now one of the most popular alternative therapies.

Properties of essential oils

Aniseed

Warming and stimulating. This oil is obtained by distillation of the seeds of the plant and is used in medical preparations to aid digestion.

Good for: nervous indigestion, migraine, asthma, bronchitis, coughs, difficulty in breathing.

Caution: do not use during pregnancy.

Basil

Uplifting and refreshing. There are many varieties of sweet basil which originated in Asia and was widely used in Indian medicine. The flowering tops and leaves are used and the oil is extracted by distillation. The leaves are heart shaped and are considered a love symbol in Italy. It is an uplifting oil which clears the head, so it makes a good nerve tonic.

Good for: indigestion, colds, sinus, migraine, muscular spasms, anxiety, depression, insomnia, asthma, catarrh, hiccups, skin problems and can be used as insect repellent.

Caution: a powerful oil, use with care.

Benzoin

Warming and relaxing. Benzoin oil is collected as a resin exuded from the trunk after the bark is cut. It is an ingredient of incense.

Good for: circulation, cystitis, rheumatoid arthritis, emotional exhaustion, tension, asthma, bronchitis, coughs, flu, chapped and cracked skin, dermatitis.

Bergamot

Uplifting and refreshing; also relaxing. The oil is obtained by expression from the fresh peel of the fruit. The fruits are somewhere between an orange and lemon in shape and change from green to yellow when ripe. Newly ripe fruits yield the best oil and half a kilo of oil is obtained from 100 kilos of fruit. Bergamot oil is a powerful antiseptic. The leaves are used in the preparation of Earl Grey tea.

Good for: indigestion, loss of appetite, cystitis, sore throat, bad breath, anxiety, depression, bronchitis, acne, psoriasis.

Caution: never use undiluted on the skin as pigmentation can occur.

Black Pepper

Stimulating. The spike of unripe berries is picked and they change from red to black as they dry in the sun. It is a green-yellow oil of great pungency.

Good for: circulation, constipation, food poisoning, indigestion, loss of appetite, colds, toothache, aches and pains, muscle tone, catarrh, coughs.

Cajuput

Antiseptic and warming. This essential oil is steam distilled from the leaves and buds of the cajuput, which grows wild in the Far East.

Good for: indigestion, cystitis, laryngitis, sinus problems, painful periods, rheumatism, aches and pains, asthma, bronchitis, tuberculosis.

Camphor

Warming and stimulating. The essential oil is present in the wood of the camphor tree.

Good for: circulation, constipation, aches and pains, rheumatism, sprains, depression, shock, acne, bruises, burns, oily skin.

Caution: do not use during pregnancy.

Caraway

Warming and stimulating. Distilled from the crushed seeds of the plant.

Good for: indigestion, arthritis, aches and pains, vertigo, pleurisy.

Cedarwood

Sedative. One of the earliest essential oils, it was used to preserve mummies. It is obtained by steam distillation from the wood. For many years it has been used by natives for medical purposes.

Good for: cystitis, anxiety, asthma, bronchitis, catarrh, coughs, acne, dandruff, irritated skin, oily skin.

Chamomile

Refreshing and relaxing. There are three similar plants with the common name chamomile. Chamomile is helpful for most disorders and is especially suitable for small children as it has low toxicity.

Good for: diarrhoea, indigestion, liver disorders, loss of appetite, stomach ulcers, headache, conjunctivitis, earache, toothache, menstrual problems, aches and pains (especially after sports), arthritis, rheumatism, anxiety, depression, insomnia, irritability, acne, allergies, broken veins, burns, dermatitis, dry scalp, eczema, inflammation.

Cinnamon

Antiseptic and digestive. It is steam distilled from both the leaves and bark of the tree.

Good for: indigestion, coughs, spots and blemishes.

Caution: skin irritant so use with care.

Clary-Sage
Warming and relaxing (aphrodisiac). The flowering tops and foliage of this plant are used to extract oil. The word 'clary'

stems from the Latin for 'clear', because an eye lotion used to be made from Clary-Sage seeds.

The oils vary widely in quality depending on what time of day the plant is picked, the dryness of the plant and whether the seeds are completely formed.

Good for: high blood pressure, sore throat, menstrual problems, depression, tension and nervous anxiety.

Clove

Antiseptic and warming. The best oil is distilled from the flower buds. The spice was highly valued in the nineteenth century.

Good for: high blood pressure, diarrhoea, indigestion, sinusitis, toothache, muscular pain, neuralgia, asthma, bronchitis, measles.

Coriander

Warming and stimulating. Coriander oil is steam distilled from the seeds. It makes an excellent stimulant of the digestive and nervous system.

Good for: indigestion, sluggish digestion, constipation, rheumatism, aches and pains, arthritis, mental fatigue.

Cypress

Relaxing and refreshing. Cypress is distilled from leaves, flowers and sometimes twigs. The oils is sometimes yellow.

Good for: prevention and treatment of cancer, circulation, chilblains, varicose veins, diarrhoea, fluid retention, laryngitis, menstrual problems, muscular cramp, irritability, asthma, oily skin, broken capillaries.

Eucalyptus

Head clearing. The oil is obtained from the fresh leaves which are rich in essential oil. Eucalyptus is one of the tallest trees in the world and trees have to be kept beheaded to make their branches more accessible. It is commonly used in chest rubs, to improve breathing in colds and sinusitis, and it has a cooling effect on body temperature.

Good for: diarrhoea, cystitis, fluid retention, colds, congestive headache, sinus problems, throat infections, aches and pains, rheumatoid arthritis, asthma, bronchitis, catarrh, flu, burns, wounds.

Fennel
Carminative (eases wind and stomach pains). Fennel has a sweet scent reminiscent of aniseed and is commonly used in cooking.

The combination of its effect on the hormones and its diuretic properties make it a valuable oil for reducing obesity. It is also renowned for its ability to aid digestive problems.

Good for: constipation, food poisoning, hiccups, indigestion, loss of appetite, cystitis, fluid retention, menstrual problems, flu prevention, hiccups, bruises, cellulite.

Caution: Use with care and not during pregnancy.

Frankincense

Relaxing and rejuvenating. This is a whitish gum which requires to be dissolved and distilled to produce essential oil.

Good for: haemorrhoids, cystitis, laryngitis, nosebleed, anxiety, depression, tension, catarrh, skin conditions.

Geranium

Refreshing and relaxing. Steam distillation is used to extract this oil from the green parts of the plant, especially the leaves.
Good for: diabetes, fluid retention, stomach ulcers, urinary tract disorders, throat and mouth infections, menstrual problems, anxiety, depression, burns, chapped and cracked skin, dermatitis, eczema, insect repellent, oily skin.

Ginger

Warming and digestive. Ginger is distilled from the roots of the plant and has excellent digestive purposes.

Good for: circulation, sluggish digestion, sore throat, muscular aches and pains, rheumatism.

Hyssop

Decongestant (respiratory). Both the leaves and blue flowers of this plant are used in distillation to obtain essential oil. It is particularly good for asthma and other respiratory problems.

Good for: low blood pressure, indigestion, loss of appetite, kidney stones, menstrual problems, calming the nerves, asthma, bronchitis, catarrh, coughs and flu, hay fever, bruises, eczema.

Caution: this is a powerful oil and should be used with care. Do not use during pregnancy.

Jasmine

Relaxing and soothing. The oil is obtained from the flowers of this plant. It is very effective on the nervous system.

Good for: pain of any kind, anxiety, apathy, depression, breathing difficulties, catarrh, skin conditions.

Juniper

Refreshing, stimulating and relaxing. Juniper oil is distilled form the dried fruits of the juniper bush. The oil is colourless or light yellow, and grows darker and thicker with age and exposure to air.

Since ancient times it has been used for its antiseptic and diuretic properties, and it is used to flavour gin.

Good for: circulation, indigestion, cystitis, fluid retention, toothache, menstrual problems, rheumatic pain, anxiety, insomnia, stress, acne, cellulite, dermatitis, eczema, oily skin.

Lavender

Refreshing, relaxing, therapeutic. This is the most used and most versatile of all the essential oils. The oil is obtained by distillation of the plant, and oil glands are embedded among tiny hairs which cover the flower, leaves and stems.

Good for: chilblains, high blood pressure, lymphatic congestion, indigestion, cystitis, fluid retention, bad breath, earache, migraine, throat infections, menstrual problems, muscular aches and pains, lack of muscle tone, rheumatism, anxiety, depression, insomnia, irritability, acne, broken capillaries, burns, cellulite, dermatitis, eczema, inflammation, oily skin, psoriasis, sun burn.

Lemon

Refreshing and stimulating. Lemon oil is obtained from the rind of the fruit.

Good for: anemia, poor circulation, high blood pressure, diabetes, stomach ulcers, kidney stones, laryngitis, mouth ulcers, colds, sinus, arthritis, rheumatism, asthma, catarrh, broken capillaries, greasy skin, insect bites, wrinkles.

Lemongrass

Toning and refreshing. Lemongrass is obtained by distillation from two species of grasses. Distillation takes place from July to January and about 100 kilos of grass are needed to yield 21kgs of oil.

The oil is the colour of dry sherry and has a lemon smell.

Good for: indigestion, gastro-enteritis, poor muscle tone, acne.

Caution: can be a skin irritant so use with care. Do not use on babies or young children.

Majoram

Warming and fortifying. Distilled from the flowering heads, this oil was grown and used in ancient times by the Egyptians.

Good for: high blood pressure, constipation, stomach spasms, headache, migraine, menstrual problems, muscular pain, rheumatism, sprains, strains, anxiety, insomnia, irritability, asthma, catarrh, bruises.

Melissa

Uplifting and refreshing. Often called the 'elixir of life', this oil has been used medicinally since the seventeenth century. It is a very cheering oil and makes a good general tonic. Obtained through distillation of the leaves and tops which contain very little essential oil. The true oil is very expensive.

Good for: high blood pressure, indigestion, colds, headache, menstrual problems, nervous tension, bee and wasp stings, skin conditions.

Myrrh

Cooling and toning. Myrrh is a gum resin which exudes from the trunk of the plant. It was used in rejuvenating facemasks during Egyptian times, and also for embalming. Myrrh is an hormonal oil and is reputed to be a sexual tonic.

Good for: circulation, indigestion, appetite loss, bad breath, mouth ulcers, inflamed respiratory tract, skin conditions.

Neroli

Ultra-relaxing. Distilled from the flowers of the bitter orange tree. It is an effective anti-depressant.

Good for: varicose veins, indigestion, pre menstrual syndrome, anxiety, depression, insomnia, shock and skin conditions.

Niaouli

Antiseptic and analgesic. This oil is distilled from the leaves.

Good for: indigestion, urinary infections, cystitis, sore throat, sinusitis, bronchitis, insect bites.

Nutmeg

Warming and digestive. The seeds of the nutmeg tree are distilled to give the essential oil.

Good for: bad breath, toothache, abdominal cramp, indigestion, gastric ulcers, muscular aches and pains, rheumatism, anxiety.

Orange

Refreshing, relaxing. Orange oil is that distilled from the peel of the fruit. It is a good digestive oil and is beneficial to the skin.

Good for: circulation, constipation, indigestion, anxiety, insomnia, acne, oily skin, stretch marks.

Origanum

Antiseptic, sedative, warming. The flowering tops and leaves are used in the distillation.

Good for: loss of appetite, sluggish digestion, muscular aches and pains, rheumatism, asthma, bronchitis, coughs, cellulite.

Patchouli

Relaxing. The oil is obtained from young leaves and dried before being steam distilled. In small quantities the oil will uplift, but larger quantities will sedate.

Good for: fluid retention, anxiety, depression, cellulite, heals chapped and cracked skin.

Peppermint
Cooling and refreshing. Peppermint oil is distilled from the leaves and flowering tops. As well as being an excellent

therapeutic oil, it is also commonly used in confectionery and toiletry.

Good for: gall stones, heartburn, indigestion, travel sickness, bad breath, headache, sinusitis, toothache, menstrual problems, shock, bronchitis, catarrh, flu, broken capillaries, inflammation, skin irritation, toxic congestion.

Petitgrain

Refreshing and relaxing. The best petitgrain is distilled from the leaves of the bitter orange tree. This oil is has an excellent balancing effect on the skin.

Good for: insomnia, apathy, irritability and skin condition.

Pine Needle

Refreshing and antiseptic. Pine oil is distilled from the needles and cones. Used widely in soaps, bath preparations and, due to its antiseptic properties, in detergents.

Good for: gall stones, cystitis, kidney problems, sinus problems, infections of the respiratory tract, asthma, bronchitis and flu.

Rose Otto
Relaxing and soothing. Having very low toxicity, yet being very powerful, this oil is a good choice for children.

Good for: poor blood circulation, liver problems, peptic ulcer, headache, menstrual problems, depression, insomnia, nervous tension, allergy, skin conditions.

Rosemary

Invigorating and refreshing. This oil is distilled from the flowering tops and leaves. It has been in therapeutic use for hundreds of years.

Good for: low blood pressure, lymphatic congestion, poor circulation, gall stones, indigestion, fluid retention, bad breath, colds, headache, menstrual problems, muscular aches and pains, arthritis, lack of muscle tone, rheumatism, sprains, stiffness, apathy, mental fatigue, mental strain, fluid retention, asthma, bronchitis, coughs, flu, cellulite, skin congestion, dandruff.

Sage

Decongestant (circulatory). The oil is extracted from leaves which are dried in the hot sun before distilling. It is a yellow oil with a camphor-.like smell.

Sage tea, taken in the last four weeks of pregnancy, can help to relieve labour pains and helps to reduce fluid retention.

Good for: low blood pressure, indigestion, laryngitis, sore throat, toothache, menstrual problems, rheumatic conditions, asthma, bronchitis, flu, skin condition.

Caution: use this powerful oil with discretion. Best not used until the last month of pregnancy, and under the direction of an aromatherapist.

Sandalwood

Relaxing. The oil is mostly in the centre of the tree, the heartwood, and the roots. The heartwood takes 30 years to become 7 cm in diameter and the oil is extracted by steam distillation.

The trees are not cut down until fully mature and showing signs of dying.

Good for: indigestion, heartburn, hiccups, nausea, cystitis, water retention, laryngitis, sore throat, depression, insomnia, bronchitis, catarrh, flu, irritated or dry skin.

Tagetes

Fungicidal. This oil should only be used well diluted as it can irritate the skin. It is very good for athlete's foot and can be used to treat psoriasis.

Good for: menstrual problems, catarrh, infection, athlete's foot and psoriasis. Caution: do not use during pregnancy.

Tea Tree

Excellent antiseptic. This oil is only produced in Australia and is steam distilled from the leaves and small branches.

Good for: indigestion, colds, sore throat, bronchitis, infected cuts and insect bites.

Red Thyme

Antiseptic. Thyme oil is obtained from the flowering tops of the plants by steam distillation.

Red Thyme is used in cooking as well as in medicine. It is a strong antiseptic and stimulates the production of white corpuscles in the blood to counter disease, and it is also an effective nerve tonic.

Good for: cystitis, colds, coughs, depression, catarrh, flu, infected cuts and boils.

Caution: irritates the skin in strong concentrations. Used with care under the direction of an aromatherapist. Do not use on babies and children.

Sweet Thyme

Antiseptic and warming. Sweet Thyme has many therapeutic properties. It is especially helpful for headaches and is gentle enough to be used with safety on young children.

Good for: cellulite, low blood pressure, diabetes, sluggish liver, cystitis, colds, headaches, sinusitis, tonsillitis, menstrual problems, muscular aches, rheumatism, anxiety, depression, asthma, bronchitis, flu, acne, verrucae and eczema.

Ylang-Ylang

Relaxing. This is obtained by distillation of the flowers.

Good for: high blood pressure, gastro-enteritis, depression, insomnia, tension and oily skin.

4

CHIROPRACTIC

Chiropractic

The word chiropractic comes from the Greek, cheir, meaning 'hands', and praktikos, meaning 'done by'. Chiropractic involves the treatment and prevention of mechanical disorders of the joints. The chiropractor will use his hands to manipulate joints and muscles to improve function, relieve pain and increase mobility. Usually the focus is on the spine, but therapists will also work on the muscles, ligaments, joints, bones and tendons.

Chiropractic is based on the theory that minor spinal displacements can cause nerve irritation, which in turn leads to disturbances of the nervous system and eventually illness. Therapists believe many problems in the joint and muscles are brought about through stress, poor posture and accidents. This therapy is beneficial for people with neck, shoulder, back and arm pain, joint problems, sports injuries, tension headaches and migraine. It is also thought that the adjustment of joints can have a positive effect on the nervous system, giving relief to conditions such as asthma, constipation and irritable bowel syndrome.

Chiropractors use a variety of techniques to stretch and relax the muscles and adjust joints. The joint is pushed beyond its normal range of movement, without damaging it, and pressure is applied. Patients feel little or no discomfort during treatment and although a disconcerting cracking sound may be heard, this is normal part of the process, caused by gas bubbles in the fluid within the joints bursting under pressure.

5

EXERCISE FOR HEALTH

Exercise for Health

Our bodies were made for activity. To remain in good health, strong and supple, with an effective circulatory and respiratory system, each of us must exercise regularly. We learn about stagnation from nature. A river that stops moving gets putrid. The same thing happens to people who stop moving. It is particularly easy to see this principle at work in our physical bodies.

Fitness does not have to involve strenuous activity. Prolonged, steady types of exercise such as golf, swimming or walking are very beneficial, and exercise programmes should include relaxation and stretching movements as well. The importance of regular exercise for health is now firmly supported by medical evidence. The metabolic rate increases, the digestive system and circulation improve, heart muscles grow stronger, and the skin takes on a healthy glow. Also, a wide range of disorders, from anxiety, depression and insomnia to obesity, diabetes and osteoporosis (thinning of the bone) improve with regular exercise.

Exercise involving steady rhythmic movement combined with periods of 0slow stretching for flexibility is a major channel to health because it is a potent force towards making use of your full potential in every area of your life. Regular, vigorous exercise increases rather than depletes your energy. Energy for movement and for your body's metabolic activities is produced in your muscle cells in little energy factories called mitochondria. It is stored here until your body needs it for a task like producing a hormone, digesting food or thinking a thought.

When you exercise regularly, over a period of months important changes take place in your cells. The number of mitochondria in each cell increases, and this creates more sites for the production of the energy compound, so it can be produced in greater quantities, much more rapidly than before. This is one of the reasons why people who take up a programme of aerobic exercise discover new reserves of vitality.

Being inactive is a serious health hazard. It can cause high blood pressure and premature aging, and result in a stiff, flabby body. In turn, these conditions are major contributors to injury and disease. No matter how well you eat, how much rest you get and how much time you spend looking after yourself, if you don't get enough exercise you cannot achieve your full potential for health and vitality. Regular exercise will improve your life in many ways. These are outlined in more detail below.

Any kind of aerobic activity which you practice at least several times a week makes you heart work more efficiently. Your heart gradually gets stronger so that it can pump more blood with less effort. There is a lot of evidence that exercise will rejuvenate you, as well as make you look better and feel firmer. Many of the so-called characteristics of aging can be prevented if you use your body enough.

Want to get lean? Then get moving. Active people not only burn calories during exercise, but their high metabolic rate burns up energy more efficiently even when resting. This is partly due to increased activity in individual cells. And steady, vigorous exercise will not increase your appetite as many people believe. In fact it decreases it and its effect is accumulative, so the longer you continue on your programme the less inclined you will be to overeat. Short-term exercisers never get their fat supplies to budge. Long-term exercisers - those who spend at least 45 minutes working out in each session and who work out at least four times a week - burn fat. After the first half hour of moderately vigorous exercise carbohydrate-derived energy in the muscles can contribute no more than half the energy needed to sustain movement, so our body is forced to begin releasing its fat stores. To take advantage of this fat burning ability you need to exercise at least three or four times a week for between 30 minutes and one hour. The enzymes that burn fat are quite different from those that burn glucose. If you are out of shape and fat, your ability to burn fat energy greatly decreases. The fitter you get, the more fat you will burn.

A high level of regular aerobic activity burns off a lot of toxic substances accumulated from food and the environment, and eliminates many harmful metabolic wastes which can cause mental and physical tension and fatigue. It also uses up a number of chemicals produced by your body when it is under stress. So it is one of the most effective methods you can find for combating the negative effects of long-term stress. It also eliminates the pressurized feeling which comes when you are worried or overworked. When you are under stress, your body produces chemicals which are designed to mobilize the body for flight or fight. But, because modern life is so sedentary, most people simply never get a chance to burn them off. For instance, excess adrenaline tends to get stored in the brain and heart, where they can affect function and alter your moods. Physical activity clears away the adrenaline build-up leaving you feeling relaxed, and restoring a healthy balance to your nervous system.

Studies of people who have taken up exercise show that some very positive psychological changes take place. They feel better about themselves and their lives. In part this is to do with biochemical changes that occur through fitness, and it can also be attributed to a change in self-image. Not only does being fit make you look leaner and firmer, it also induces a state of consciousness which is more positive and it dramatically alters you whole outlook on life, bringing a sense of long term well-being. When you feel good and positive about yourself it is easy to choose foods which are good for you and you tend to leave behind bad habits. You simply don't want or need them any more.

The biochemical explanation for the kind of positive emotional and mental changes fitness brings seem to be related to messenger chemicals called neurotransmitters. These carry powerful implications for mental clarity and moods. The hormone noradrenaline is known for its ability to lift our mood and to lessen feelings of discomfort and fatigue. People with sunny dispositions tend to have high levels of noradrenaline in their bloodstream, while depressed people have low levels. Vigorous exercise increases the production of noradrenaline. This is probably one of the reasons why so many emotional disorders, from anxiety to depression, have been successfully treated with exercise.

There are now an abundance of well-established reasons why exercise is good for you.
increased energy and stamina
less fat tissue and increased lean muscle tissue, which burns calories efficiently (nothing is burnt by fat tissue)
improved use of nutrients from the food we eat
more restful sleep
improved self-image, more attractive looks, a more positive attitude to life
slowing of the aging process
healthier skin with fewer wrinkles
So do it!

6

FLOWER REMEDIES

Flower remedies

Flower remedies are used to alleviate emotional and stress related conditions. Flowers are picked at the peak of their blossoming and put in glass containers holding distilled water for about three hours. The flowers are then discarded and the water preserved in brandy. This is the mother tincture from which most of the Flower Remedies are prepared. They are not used directly for physical problems, rather the emphasis is on balancing the emotions so that the body is free to heal itself. The remedies are used for a variety of emotions. In particular there is the Rescue Remedy, a mixture of five remedies designed to comfort, reassure and calm after a severe upset or serious bad news.

Flower remedies are usually attributed to Edward Bach. Born in 1887, he was a doctor, bacteriologist and later a homeopath. His intention was to develop a method of healing which would treat the emotional and spiritual imbalances which lead to physical disease. He believed that flower essences could be used to positively affect people's moods and state of mind, and hence have a therapeutic effect on their health. Flower remedies can also be extracted from the flowers of wild plants, bushes and trees through soaking the flower heads in spring water in the sun for several hours or by boiling the woody plants. The resulting mixture is preserved in brandy and taken internally to lift the spirits. The principle of this therapy is the strong link between emotions and our physical condition.

Dr Bach devised 36 remedies in total, which in combination are believed to cover all possible states of mind. Each of the remedies acts on a negative emotional state to induce its corresponding positive side. They are as follows;

Fear
Aspen-acts on fear of the unknown.

Red Chestnut- acts on excessive concern for the welfare of others.

Cherry Plum- acts on desperation arising from fear of losing control.

Rock Rose- acts on terror or panic, total self-involvement or self abandonment. Brings the ability to act selflessly.

Mimulus- acts on fear of known things, shyness and speech impediments that arise form lack of trust in a divine pattern. Promotes faith and courage, acceptance and endurance.

Uncertainty
Gorse- acts on feeling of hopelessness.

Hornbeam- acts on tiredness caused by self doubt.

Wild Oats- acts on lack of ambition and direction.

Cerato- acts on self-distrust and the tendency to seek advice form others. It promotes self-reliance, intuitiveness and qualities of leadership.

Scleranthus- acts on indecision, mood swings and motion sickness. It promotes stability and decisiveness.

Gentian- acts on discouragement and disappointments that produce reactive depression. It promotes optimism and perseverance.

Lack of interest. (In the present.)
Clematis- acts on dreaminess, escapism and absentmindedness. It promotes alertness

Honeysuckle- acts on nostalgia and suffering from the loss of a person or object that you love.

Wild Rose- acts on resignation and feelings of apathy.

Olive- acts on the effects of physical and mental stress.

White Chestnut- acts on a preoccupation with persistent, unwanted worrying thoughts.

Chestnut Bud- acts on the tendency to repeat mistakes, to be slow to learn from experience.

Loneliness.
Water Violet- acts on excessive self-sufficiency.

Heather- acts on excessive self-concern, talkativeness, and a dislike of being alone.

Impatiens- acts on impatience, instability and accident proneness.

Over sensitivity. (to influence and ideas.)
Walnut- acts on over sensitivity to outside influences and is helpful for the major changes in life such as puberty and the menopause.

Holly- acts on anger or hatred, generally when they are directed against others, but also when self-directed.

Agrimony- acts on worry or mental torment concealed by a mask of happiness or sociability.

Centaury- acts on an inability to say no and an excessive anxiety to please. Those who need Centaury tend to bottle up anger and depression.

Depression and anguish.

Mustard- acts on sudden deep depression with no known cause.

Larch- acts on lack of confidence and fear of failure.

Pine- acts on guilt, both real and imagined, and the tendency to apologize needlessly.

Elm- acts on a sudden feeling of being overwhelmed by responsibility.

Sweet Chestnut- acts on extreme anguish and a feeling of total bereavement.

Star of Bethlehem- relieves the effects of any type of shock.

Willow- acts on resentment and bitterness.

Oak- acts on a tendency to relentless effort which can lead to a breakdown of mind or body, especially back problems.

Crab Apple- relieves feelings of uncleanness.

Over concern. (for the welfare of others.)

Chicory- acts on a tendency to take over people or situations.

Vervain- moderates extremes of energy, tension and enthusiasm.

Vine- corrects a tendency to extreme control of yourself or of others, and excess will.

Beech- corrects a tendency to intolerance and criticism of others.

Rock Water- corrects excessive self-involvement, leading to mental rigidity.

Rescue Remedy. A mixture of Impatiens, Star of Bethlehem, Cherry Plum, Rock Rose and Clematis. Is very effective whenever there is a combination of shock and panic, faintness or hysteria, for example, after an accident or other trauma or before a stressful event such as an exam. Keep it handy, and take it as required, every few minutes if necessary, until you feel calm and in control.

7

FOOD FOR HEALTH

Food for Health

Between 50 000 and 100 000 different chemicals go into the making and running of the human body. They interact with each other in ways so complex that they make the world's most advanced computer look like an abacus. Complex chemical transformations take place in our bodies every minute of every day and these require a variety of quality nutrients. That's why changes in diet profoundly affect how we look and feel, and for many of us that is the most important proof that what we are doing is right for us.

Overeating, processed foods, under-exercising, stress and pollution are some of the most common and most dangerous elements of the late twentieth century. It is hardly surprising that a lifestyle which deviates so far from what our bodies over millions of years have been genetically programmed to expect leads to lack of vitality, illness and disease. The body has extraordinary powers of compensation and for many years one can eat the wrong foods, take little exercise and overwork without showing clinical signs of illness. But the degenerative process is at work and sooner or later hidden degeneration turns into serious problems.

The immune system protects the body from infection, malignant growths and early aging. Studies show that the nutrients which occur in fresh uncooked vegetables strengthen the immune system and increase resistance to disease. The nutrients that most favourably influence the immune system are vitamins E, C and A, and many of the B vitamins and also zinc. Health and fitness depend largely on the quality and variety of the nutrients we take in, and a full complement of fresh food nutrients is essential for optimum immunity to be maintained.

Foods in nature are highly complex, rich in structural information for health. Cooking and other forms of processing interfere with this complexity and destroy much of this structural information. For the body to function at its full potential the substances supplied to sustain it must be in the same mixtures and concentrations that occur in raw, unprocessed foods. Food should be as close to its natural state as possible, as evolution has designed our mechanisms precisely to deal with it in this way.

The health promoting effects that unprocessed and uncooked foods have on the body are such that a largely fresh, raw diet slows the rate at which you age, gives you lots of energy and even makes you feel better emotionally. Scientists involved in raw food research and in the treatment of illness using raw food diets believe that many people are living in a state of half-hearted health induced by years of eating devitalised and processed foods. Though there has been a strong swing away from meat and fat towards fiber and fresh foods, most people in Britain continue to exist on a diet high in cooked and processed foods.

Research carried out by Paul Kouchakoff at the Institute of Clinical Chemistry in Lousanne in the 1930's gives an interesting theory on the effects of cooked food. What his work implies is that the body identifies cooked and processed foods as harmful invaders and tries to wipe them out as it would bacteria or a virus. So when cooked or processed foods are eaten, white blood cells (leucocytes) rush to the intestine.

This phenomenon is called 'digestive leucocytosis', and before Kouchakoff's research it was thought to be a normal part of the digestive process. But Kouchakoff discovered that when food is eaten raw, digestive leucocytosis does not take place. When his volunteers ate raw food, the number of white blood cells in the bloodstream did not increase, yet processed and cooked food reliably triggered off white cell mobilisation. Interestingly leucocytosis does not take place if raw food is eaten before cooked food.

The implications of leucocytosis are as follows. Each time white blood cells rush to the intestines to deal with cooked food the rest of the body is left undefended against germs, virus and disease. Continual red alerts, three or more times a day, year in year out, put an enormous strain on the immune system. Raw foods leave the white blood cells free for other tasks and save the body the effort of a defensive action, thereby strengthening the body's resistance to disease. The healing and health promoting properties of uncooked foods are widely recognised in natural therapies. Uncooked diets combined with other natural methods of healing and exercise are used to treat all kinds of illness. The basis of the biological approach is the belief that sickness is the result of disturbances in the body's natural chemistry and that once these disturbances are corrected the body's own healing forces, which are very powerful, can deal with the cause.

Our health is dependent on the constant interchange of chemicals and energy between the bloodstream and the cells. The bloodstream, via the capillaries, supplies the tissues of the body with oxygen and nutrients and carries away cellular waste. This interchange of chemicals and energy occurs because cells and capillaries attract the substances they need and reject what is harmful or unnecessary. This attraction and rejection is the result of antagonistic chemical and micro electrical tensions between cells in a living system. When you die it is lost completely. The stronger the tensions, the more intense these antagonisms, the healthier and more vital your body will be. At the University of Vienna scientists showed that raw food heightens electrical potentials between tissue cells and capillary blood. This improves the capillaries ability to regulate the transportation of nutrients, and gradually detoxifies the system.

Over quite a short time a high raw diet does several things.

⇒It eliminates accumulated wastes and toxins.

⇒It restores acid/alkaline balance.

⇒It supplies the level of nutrients necessary for optimal cell function.

⇒It increases the efficiency with which cells take up oxygen, which in turn improves the cells' ability to carry out their many activities.

⇒It makes us feel and look great.

No one would question that cooked foods have the ability to sustain life. What is questioned by doctors and scientists involved in research into raw diets is whether cooked foods are capable of regenerating and enhancing health. Experiments and studies have revealed that food processing and cooking, particularly at high temperatures, brings about changes in the nature of food proteins, fats and fiber which not only make them less health promoting to the body, but may even make them harmful.

Cooking also damages the vitamins in our food. Vitamins are organic substances which the body requires in very small amounts to carry out its thousands of building up and breaking down operations. Some vitamins, such as vitamin

D, can be manufactured by the body, but most are obtained from food. Many of these vital vitamins are destroyed by cooking. Vitamin C and the B vitamins are water soluble, which makes them particularly vulnerable. Not only are they very sensitive to heat, but they leach out when food is soaked, blanched or boiled. Putting a cabbage into cold water and bringing it to the boil destroys 75% of its vitamin C content. Cooking fresh peas for five minutes wipes out 20-40% of their thiamin (one of the B vitamins) and 30-40% of their vitamin C. Fresh milk contains 10% more vitamins and 15% more vitamin C than milk which has been pasteurised at high temperatures. Vitamins A, D, E and K are fat-soluble and therefore less at risk, remaining relatively stable up to about 212 degrees f (boiling point of water). However, up to 50% of the vitamin E content in food may be destroyed by frying or baking. Vital vitamins are lost in the preserving and canning process as well.

Raw protein boosts our health also. A protein is a chain of amino acids of which there are around twenty known in nature. Strung together in special sequences amino acids make up all the proteins there are. Eight to ten of these appear to be essential for our nutrition, and out bodies need these almost all of the time. When proteins are heated some of these amino acids become changed in their molecular structure, and some amino acids are destroyed completely. If you grill steak to 239 degrees f, the amino acids cystine and lysine are lost. Glutamine, which is believed to help arthritis, can also be destroyed by heat. Damaging protein by cooking means we need to eat more of it to get the amino acids we need. This is risky considering that too much protein appears to be detrimental to health in general and is especially implicit in cancer. Too much protein leads to deficiencies of the B vitamins niacin and B6, calcium, magnesium and other minerals, and also puts enormous strain on the pancreas, the organ responsible for manufacturing the enzymes needed to digest protein. The same enzymes that digest protein are also thought to prevent our bodies from cancer. Many scientists believe consider the loss of pancreatic function to be a major cause of cancer. It is therefore important to save most of the enzymes the pancreas produces for combating malignancy rather than digesting protein.

When fats are heated to high temperatures the molecular structure of their fatty acids changes. Analysis of heated oils shows they contain numerous poisonous compounds which can cause damage to the structure of cell membranes, cell nuclei and proteins. That's why we should not fry food at high temperatures, or reheat cooking oil. In the heating process (used to make margarine, cooking oil, and many convenience foods) valuable 'cis' fatty acids, which the body needs and can make use of are converted into 'trans' fatty acids, which the body cannot use. That is why it is possible to eat a lot of fat and still fail to get the fatty acids you need. Recent research indicates that many people do suffer from fatty acid deficiency. So try to include unheated extra virgin olive oil in your diet. It is a valuable source of the fatty acids your body needs, it's non- toxic, and it makes a delicious salad dressing into the bargain. If you are going to fry food, olive oil is probably the safest as it only contains four fatty acids, but it should never be heated to smoking point.

Perhaps the most important of the health giving raw plant factors are the enzymes. Enzymes are the essential triggers for the metabolic machinery of every living thing. Some are extraordinarily powerful. For example, the pepsin produced in your stomach breaks down the white of an egg in just a few minutes, but it takes 24 hours to achieve this in a laboratory. There are tens of thousands of enzymes working away in your body, breaking down food and assimilating it, building new tissue and repairing it and manufacturing more enzymes so that the essential work can continue. We grow old when enough metabolic errors accumulate to injure the production of our enzymes. Many practitioners maintain that raw foods are important because they help support the body's own enzyme systems. They believe that each food contains exactly the amount of enzymes, vitamins and minerals required to help break down that particular food. Enzymes are completely destroyed by cooking, and when we eat cooked food our body has to make more of its own digestive enzymes to properly digest and assimilate them. Without the enzymes from raw foods your body's own enzyme production abilities tend to wane as the years pass by. By eating a diet high in raw food you ensure that your body has an outside supply of enzymes which will help you to live longer, have more energy, look more youthful and stay healthier.

8

Food properties

Alfafa

- One of the richest sources of potassium, iron, zinc, magnesium, phosphorus and calcium. Of all plants it is richest in chlorophyll (2%).
- Contains vitamins A, B, D, E, G, C, and vitamin K which your body needs to clot blood.
- Rich in essential amino acids.
- Contains sterole, which produces sex hormones.
- Strong alkalizing effect, which can help to restore the internal acid/alkali balance.
- High in protein.

Natural therapeutic properties
digestive, laxative, diuretic, tonic

Beneficial for treating
⇒weak immune system
⇒hard arteries
⇒anaemia
⇒arthritis

⇒kidney inflammation

Almonds

- Can be used as a substitute for meat or milk as almonds are high in protein (21%)
- Rich in calcium, phosphorus, manganese, potassium, magnesium, iron and vitamin A

Natural therapeutic properties
- sedative, tonic

Beneficial for treating
⇒asthma and skin conditions which can be provoked by dairy products
⇒diabetes
⇒colon and bowel problems
⇒kidney disease
⇒muscle and bone weakness

Aniseed

- Helps digestion
- Can be used to balance the effects of coffee

Natural therapeutic properties
diuretic, relieves flatulence, digestive, stimulant, tonic, expectorant

Beneficial for treating

⇒poor digestion

⇒flatulence

⇒cramps

⇒colic

⇒nausea

Apples

- Rich in potassium, sodium, vitamin A, B1 and vitamin C
- Plentiful source of phosphorus (a valuable brain food) which helps you to think clearly
- High in minerals (3-4g in every litre)

Natural therapeutic properties

cleansing

Beneficial for treating

⇒sluggish digestion

⇒burns - a slice of raw apple placed immediately on a burn will prevent blistering

⇒arthritis - apples are rich in malic and citric acid which help to neutralize too much acidity in the blood

⇒kidney problems - apples contain potassium salts which act as a diuretic

⇒kidney stones

⇒hypertension - apples reduce our sodium content which in turn reduces hypertension and blood pressure

Apricots

- Rich in potassium, sodium, magnesium, B17 and iron
- Contain a high concentration of beta carotene

Natural therapeutic properties
healing, tonic

Beneficial for treating
⇒constipation
⇒cancer

Avocados
- Highest vitamin E content of any fruit
- Rich in proteins, phosphorus, sulphur and chlorine
- High content of copper, iron, potassium and sodium
- Contain everything our body requires, except for vitamin C

Beneficial for treating
⇒digestive complaints
⇒halitosis
⇒gall bladder disease

Bananas

- Rich in calcium, magnesium, potassium, phosphorus, sulphur, copper and iron
- Contains vitamins A, B, C and E.

Natural therapeutic properties
digestive

Beneficial for treating
⇒stomach ulcers - bananas neutralize the stomach acid and thicken the mucus lining in the stomach

⇒anaemia

⇒diabetes - bananas contain a high content of easily absorbed sugars

⇒high blood cholesterol - due to the pectin content

Beans

- Rich in proteins
- Contains iron, zinc, potassium, calcium and phosphorus

Natural therapeutic properties
diuretic, anti-cancer

Beneficial for treating
⇒high cholesterol

⇒cancer - research indicates beans may prevent cancer because they contain isoflovones, which act as a protective shield against invading cells

⇒rheumatism

⇒kidney and urinary problems

Beetroot

- Rich in potassium, sodium, calcium, magnesium, phosphorus, sulphur, silicon and iron
- High in vitamin A

Natural therapeutic properties
nerve tonic, rebuilds blood cells

Beneficial for treating
⇒calcium deposits

⇒heart troubles attributed to thickening arteries

⇒varicose veins

⇒liver and kidney disease

⇒gallstones

⇒anaemia

Blackcurrants

- Contains anthocyanosides (these destroy the bacteria E coli that cause diarrhoea)

Natural therapeutic properties
astringent, tonic

Beneficial for treating
⇒diarrhoea
⇒appendicitis
⇒high blood cholesterol

Broccoli

- Contains vitamin A, beta carotene, vitamin C, zinc and potassium
- High in chlorophyll

Natural therapeutic properties
anti-cancerous, anti-catarrhal, strengthens the immune system

Beneficial for treating
⇒anaemia
⇒cancer

Cabbage

- Rich in sulphur
- Contains vitamins U, C

Beneficial for treating
(for best results use raw cabbage juice)

⇒gout

⇒rheumatism

⇒ulcers

⇒spots and blisters

⇒headache

⇒burns

⇒asthma

⇒cystitis

⇒bronchitis

Carrots

- Contains large amounts of beta carotene
- Rich in vitamin A, potassium, sulphur, sodium, phosphorus and iron
- Contains vitamins B, C and E
- Contains large doses of calcium

Natural therapeutic properties
diuretic, stimulant

Beneficial for treating
(Raw carrots are most potent)

⇒failing eyesight

⇒poor complexion

⇒colds

⇒nervous conditions

⇒anaemia

⇒cancer

Cauliflower

- Rich in sulphur

Natural therapeutic properties
anti-cancerous

Beneficial for treating
⇒cancer

⇒ulcers - if taken in juice form in combination with potato juice

⇒arthritis - should be applied as a poultice

Celery

- Rich in zinc, sodium, potassium and sulphur
- Contains vitamins A and G

Natural therapeutic properties
anti-inflammatory, ant-arthritic, blood purifying, digestive

Beneficial for treating
(Most effective used in fresh juice form)

⇒arthritis - the high sodium content helps prevent crystal formation

⇒liver problems

⇒high blood pressure

Cider vinegar

- Packed full of essential amino acids, vitamins, minerals and enzymes
- Rich in pectin

Natural therapeutic properties
preservative, cure-all

Beneficial for treating
(Take internally, 3 teaspoons with one tablespoon honey in a cup of hot water)

⇒infection

⇒varicose veins

⇒acidity

⇒headaches

⇒sore throats

⇒calcium deposits

⇒excessive appetite

⇒memory loss

Caution
Cider and fermented apple juice can suppress the body's ability to dissolve blood clots. Fresh apples do not have this effect

Cucumber

- Rich in potassium, phosphorus, iron, silicon and calcium

Natural therapeutic properties
diuretic, laxative

Beneficial for treating
⇒ulcers
⇒poor digestion

Garlic

- Contains vitamins B, C and A
- Rich in calcium, sulphur, zinc, copper, potassium and phosphoric acid

Natural therapeutic properties
stimulant, aphrodisiac, tonic, diuretic, anti-bacterial, antioxidant

Beneficial for treating
⇒high blood cholesterol
⇒weak immune system
⇒digestive problems
⇒pneumonia and tuberculosis
⇒bronchitis
⇒catarrh

Ginger

- Contains gingerol which has similar painkilling and blood thinning properties to aspirin.

Natural therapeutic properties
appetizing, stimulant, antioxidant, anti-coagulant

Beneficial for treating
⇒colic

⇒vomiting

⇒travel sickness - such a thick slice of ginger without chewing

Grapes

- Immensely valuable healing fruit
- Contains large amounts of potassium
- Rich in glucose which strengthens the heart and its muscles
- Contains vitamins A, B1, B2 and C
- Contains tartaric acid which stimulates the intestines

Natural therapeutic properties
laxative, cooling, diuretic

Beneficial for treating
⇒kidney troubles

⇒anaemia
⇒rheumatism and arthritis

Honey (must be cold pressed without additives)

- Has outstanding antiseptic properties
- Heals burns without leaving scar tissue
- Withdraws moisture from bacteria, causing them to die

Natural therapeutic properties
antiseptic, tonic

Beneficial for treating
⇒athlete's foot - apply direct to the affected area
⇒cuts
⇒burns
⇒throat infections

Lemons

- Rich in vitamins B and C
- High in potassium
- Lemons destroy bacteria without damaging body tissue

Natural therapeutic properties
antiseptic, anti-acid, antifungal

Beneficial for treating
⇒gastric complaints

⇒piles

⇒boils

⇒asthma

⇒diabetes

⇒catarrh

⇒anaemia

Onions

- Helps to combat colds and coughs
- Contains large amounts of vitamins A and E which guard against free radical
- Rich in vitamin C, calcium, iron and sulphur
- Powerful healer

Natural therapeutic properties
antioxidant, antifungal, antibacterial, anti-cancerous, antiseptic, antispasmodic, diuretic, expectorant, digestive, tonic

Beneficial for treating
⇒catarrh

⇒anaemia

⇒coughs and colds

⇒influenza

⇒liver cirrhosis

⇒kidney diseases

⇒tuberculosis

⇒bronchitis

⇒insomnia

⇒toothache

⇒bruises

⇒anxiety

Oranges

- Rich source of mineral salts, especially calcium
- Rich source of vitamins, especially vitamin C
- Strongly alkaline forming

Beneficial for treating

⇒fevers

⇒colds

⇒excessive stomach acidity

Oysters

- Rich in zinc - making them a strong aphrodisiac, especially for men
- Abundant supply of omega 3 fatty acids - these help to lower cholesterol
- Rich in amino acid

- One of the purest protein foods

Natural therapeutic effects
blood-purifying, aphrodisiac, good for kidneys

Beneficial for treating
⇒insomnia
⇒rheumatoid arthritis
⇒asthma
⇒allergies
⇒psoriasis
⇒cancer
⇒eating disorders
⇒heart problems

Papaya

- Richer in vitamin A than cod liver oil
- Good source of calcium
- Strongly alkaline

Natural therapeutic properties
Digestive, healing

Beneficial for treating
⇒liver problems
⇒constipation

⇒flatulence

Peaches
- Rich in iron
- Alkaline

Beneficial for treating
⇒anaemia
⇒indigestion
⇒intestinal disorders
⇒blood impurities

Peppercorns

- Kill germs and bacteria
- Outer skin is anticatarrhal

Natural therapeutic properties
aromatic, stimulant, digestive, nerve tonic, diuretic

Beneficial for treating
⇒catarrh - coarse black pepper should be used as it contains
   the skin which helps prevent catarrh
⇒sore throats
⇒colds involving sneezing

Pineapples

- Remove uric acid from our system
- Contains bromelaine which helps to digest proteins in meat, fish, milk and egg whites

Natural therapeutic properties
anti-arthritic, anti-rheumatic

Beneficial for treating
⇒heart and kidney disease
⇒overworked kidneys

Caution
Unripe pineapples may cause mouth ulcers

Plums

- Rich in calcium, phosphorus, iron and potassium
- Good source of vitamins A, B and C

Natural therapeutic properties
astringent, laxative

Beneficial for treating
⇒Irritability - plums work directly on the nervous system and can be very uplifting
⇒Constipation

Potatoes

- Highly alkaline
- Rich in vitamins A and B
- Skin contains chlorogenic acid which helps to prevent cancer

Natural therapeutic properties
anti-inflammatory, anti-ulcerous

Beneficial for treating
⇒heart disease
⇒high blood pressure
⇒tooth decay
⇒rheumatism
⇒hardening of the arteries
⇒constipation

Caution
Do not eat potatoes that have sprouted, they contain solanin which is harmful

Raspberries

- Strengthen the immune system
- Highly alkaline
- Rich in iron

- Source of vitamin C

Natural therapeutic properties
astringent, laxative

Beneficial for treating
⇒fevers
⇒rheumatism
⇒joint aches and pain

Spinach

- Rich in zinc, calcium, iron, manganese, copper, iodine and chlorophyll
- Abundant source of vitamin A, and also contains vitamins B, C and D
- Alkaline

Natural therapeutic properties
blood builder, lung protector, eye-strengthener, alkaline-forming

Beneficial for treating
(for best results use spinach juice)
⇒night-blindness
⇒bleeding gums
⇒constipation
⇒glandular disturbances

⇒obesity

⇒high or low blood pressure

⇒rheumatism

⇒eye diseases

⇒nervous exhaustion

⇒migraine

⇒sore throats

Strawberries

- Contain large amounts of kalium
- Rich in vitamins A and C
- Good source of iron
- Good source of pectin

Natural therapeutic properties
Anti-viral, anti-cancerous

Beneficial for treating
⇒gout

⇒rheumatism

Tomatoes
- Rich source of vitamins A, B and C
- Rich in minerals, especially magnesium
- High iron content - contains twice as much as milk

Natural therapeutic properties
alkalizing, cleanses the blood, kidney tonic

Beneficial for treating
⇒premature aging
⇒sluggish liver
⇒bronchitis
⇒asthma

Watercress
- Rich in iron, phosphates and potassium
- Contains iodine and sulphur
- Good source of vitamins A and C

Natural therapeutic properties
diuretic, expectorant, stimulant, digestive

Beneficial for treating
⇒headaches
⇒asthma
⇒coughs
⇒sleeplessness

Watermelons
- Rich in vitamins A, B and C
- Good source of minerals
- Remedy for all kidney problems

Natural therapeutic properties
diuretic

Beneficial for treating
⇒kidney problems
⇒kidney stones

Yams (sweet potatoes)

• High in beta carotene

Natural therapeutic properties
Support eye and lung function

Beneficial for treating
⇒pre-menstrual syndrome
⇒diarrhoea
⇒coughs
⇒asthma
⇒kidney disease
⇒diabetes

.

9

HERBAL MEDICINE

Herbal Medicine

Herbal medicine is one of the oldest forms of medicine in the world, and until the late nineteenth century, all medicines were derived form plants. As medicine became more scientific, scientists learned how to isolate active ingredients in the plants and synthesise them in laboratories. Herbalists argue that the balance achieved in nature cannot be reproduced in a test-tube. They believe that the whole plant must be used to treat the patient as the balance of elements prevents side effects.

Herbal medicine is taken as herbal tinctures, which are herbs in alcohol and water, or syrups, made by boiling the herb in water and adding sugar as a preservative. Herbalists may also administer the herbs in the form of teas, poultices or ointments and the usually give advice on diet and lifestyle too. This therapy is thought to build up the body's defences so that the body can fight off illness and heal itself.

Many people are fiercely loyal to herbal medicine. Around 5 million people in Britain regularly buy herbal remedies and there are around 1,500 herbalists. Herbal medicine was established formally in Britain by an act of parliament during the reign of Henry VIII.

Alternative medicine on the whole is also booming. There are more than 4 million visits each year to alternative therapists, and the number of therapists in the UK is increasing annually by around 11%. Growing awareness of the benefits of alternative medicine and fitness combined with dissatisfaction towards conventional medicine and its associated limitations and side affects are having a profound effect on the popularity of alternative medicine. More clinics than ever are now offering holistic health care in response to this surging public demand for non-toxic, natural, health boosting medical care.

The primary goal of alternative medicine is firstly to identify the cause of the illness, and then to change any lifestyle factors (such as an unsuitable diet, not enough exercise, or too much alcohol) which may be making the problems worse, and then to cure it through stimulation of the body's natural healing response, which is extremely powerful. Most prescribed drug treatments merely mask symptoms and do not address the origins of the illness. Alternative medicine works in two ways. It is both preventative and curative. It promotes good health and a strong immune system which helps prevent illness and disease. And it cures existing ill health through tackling the root cause of the problem.

10

HOMEOPATHY

Homeopathy

Homeopathy is a therapeutic method of medicine consisting of very dilute doses of natural substances. It works on the principle that tiny doses of these substances cure the same symptoms which strong doses of the same substance actually cause. Despite dating back 500 BC to the Greek physician, Hippocrates, aromatherapy only became widely known in the eighteenth century when it was rediscovered by a German physician, Hahnemann. He observed that although cinchona bark produced malaria type fevers, when tiny doses of the cinchona were given to patients, their malaria fevers were reduced.

Homeopathy stimulates the body's own defences to correct illness. The word homeopathy originates from the Greek homoios, meaning 'like' and pathos, meaning 'suffering'. The therapy is based on an ancient principle 'let like be treated by like', and the cure of the illness is achieved by treating patients with a substances which mimics the illness.

A homeopath will take into consideration all aspects of the health of an individual, including the emotional and mental state of the patient, before prescribing a remedy specifically targeted to stimulate the body's recuperative powers. Homeopathic remedies can be in the form of tablets, granules, powder or liquid which the patient takes by mouth, or in the form of creams and drops. They are prepared by taking a solution of the concentrated ingredient and diluting it. At each stage of the dilution the preparation is shaken vigorously. Homeopaths believe that this vigorous shaking is important to achieve the therapeutic effect of the solution. Ironically, the more diluted the solution the more effective it is.

Homeopathy is suitable for a wide range of conditions, such as hay fever, asthma, irritable bowel syndrome, eczema, and premenstrual tension. It is particularly beneficial where there is an emotional link to the illness, such as recent bereavement or stress. It is also used to alleviate chronic diseases such as rheumatoid arthritis, which are thought to be caused by the body attacking itself because the immune system has somehow become confused. Homeopathic medicine is believed to give the body new and correct information, allowing it to heal itself.

Some of those who try homeopathy feel an immediate improvement, while others may require treatment over a number of months. Homeopaths subscribe to the rule that one month's treatment is required for every year the person has had the illness. A homeopathic remedy is specific to a particular person at a particular time. Therapists believe that everyone has a unique personal energy and a pattern of susceptibility to illness and other influences. By closely matching remedies to the individual, homeopaths balance these energy patterns and restore health.

Homeopathy can be traced back to the fourth century BC, to the Greek physician, Hippocrates, but it was a German doctor, Samuel Hahnemann, who formulated the principle for the modern world in the late eighteenth century. He trained in orthodox medicine, but became disillusioned with it and began to experiment with other ways of healing. He published the Law of Similars in 1796. In the mid-nineteenth century homeopathy gained popularity, and during the cholera epidemic of 1845 the London Homeopathic Hospital was renowned for having a death rate of only 16%, compared to 60% in general hospitals.

11

NATUROPATHY

Naturopathy

The principle behind naturopathy is the simple belief that the body has the power to heal itself, given the right set of circumstances. Naturopaths believe that disease occurs due to an imbalance in the body. The aim of the naturopath is to bring the body back to the point where it can heal itself. They are not solely concerned with alleviating symptoms, rather they endeavor to correct the basic causes of disease, beginning with the principle that pure water, fresh air, exercise and a balanced diet of fresh foods are the foundations for good health. Practitioners are also skilled in soft tissue techniques, including massage and manipulation, to ease muscle tension and imbalances.

One of the main aims of the naturopath is to encourage the detoxification process. Our body is exposed to a wide variety of harmful compounds through the chemical-laden processed food we eat, and pollution in the air and water. When we take in too many of these toxins the liver, which breaks them down, is overloaded. Naturopaths may use fasting to detoxify the body, and all practitioners recommend a diet that includes plenty of fruit, preferably organic no sugar or refined foods, small amounts of free-range meat and the minimum of alcohol, tea and coffee.

Naturopaths believe that symptoms of illness are the outward signs of the body's efforts to overcome germs and viruses, and that they should not be suppressed unless they pose a serious threat to the health of the patient. For example, a naturopath would not recommend suppressing the symptoms of a cold with antibiotics, but would encourage the expulsion of the germs through the natural defensive measures (symptoms) your body automatically employs to aid its recovery.

The roots of naturopathy can be traced back 2,000 years to the Greek physician Hippocrates, who was one of the first to recognise nature's own healing powers. The ancient Greeks had temples of healing, often constructed near mineral or thermal springs, where patients were treated to a regime of bathing, exercise, massage and fasting. Modern day practitioners may also prescribe hot and cold baths, sometimes filled with epsom salts or seaweed.

12

OSTEOPATHY

Osteopathy

Osteopathy originates from the Greek words osteo (meaning bone) and pathos (meaning disease). This form of treatment was founded in the 1870's by an American doctor, Andrew Taylor Still. He believed that to be healthy, the body has to be mechanically sound, so that its self-healing mechanisms can function normally. According to the principles of osteopathy, poor health and even disease can result from imbalances in the normal tension of the spine, which affect the nervous system and result in discomfort or malfunction throughout the body.

This therapy has been practiced in Britain for over a hundred years to relieve back and joint pain, and to treat sprains, sports injuries, headaches and the discomfort of pregnancy. Osteopaths diagnose and treat the patient by manipulating the bones, joints, muscles, ligaments and connective tissues. It is directed towards freeing the joints, muscles and soft tissues, and patients generally find treatment pleasant and relaxing. Osteopaths use a variety of techniques, including massage to relax stiff muscles, stretching to increase joint mobility, and manipulation and thrust techniques to restore easy movement to the body. The treatment may also include advice on posture, diet, lifestyle or stress management.

Cranial osteopathy is an 'indirect technique' which is used to help relieve sinus problems, headaches and neuralgia. It is based on the concept that there are tiny gaps between the eight sections of the human skull. It is believed that these sections can be pushed out of position (for example, at birth or as a result of head injury) causing tension, disturbances and tissue immobility, not only in the skull itself, but also throughout the whole body. Light touching and gentle manipulation are used to ease the parts of the skull back into place, thereby reducing tension and restoring balance.

13

REFLEXOLOGY

Reflexology

In reflexology, pressure points on the feet are stimulated by the therapist. All the body's organs, parts and systems can be related to specific areas in the feet, and by massaging the feet, therapists stimulate the corresponding organs in the body, freeing blockages and releasing natural healing powers.

Foot pressure point massage is an ancient Indian and Chinese therapy which was used 5, 000 years ago. It was revived and developed by Dr William Fitzgerald, an American surgeon, in 1913 when he discovered that pressure to certain parts of the foot could ease pain in other parts of the body. He followed the belief that the body is divided into ten zones through which energy flows. These zones run from the feet, up the body to the head and down to the hands. By working on pressure points on the feet, blockages in the body which may be contributing to ill health are freed, the energy balance is corrected and a state of health is restored. Many believe that these pressure points are the same as acupuncture points. Reflexology was further advanced by a therapist called Eunice Ingham who developed a method of massaging the feet, which is the basis of the treatment as we know it today.

Reflexologists believe that crystalline deposits of calcium and uric acid build up at the nerve endings, and these can be detected as crunchy areas under the skin. This tends to indicate a weakness in the corresponding area of the body. Gentle pressure on these deposits is thought to cause them to break down and encourage the healing process to begin.

Reflexology is used to enhance energy levels and improve emotional well-being. It serves to alleviate migraine, headaches, back problems and is good for asthma, skin disorders, high blood pressure, poor circulation, constipation and irritable bowel syndrome. In any stress related conditions reflexology is thought to provide a relaxing way to restore vitality and balance, and from being an old folk medicine, it has now been developed into a skillful manual therapy which gives relief and benefit to many in today's stressful society.

Practitioners work over all areas of the feet. Initially, gentle massage is used, followed by deep thumb and finger pressure. If an imbalance or blockage is present, the area of the foot which corresponds to the affected body part may feel tender, and gentle pressure is used to remove the blockage.

14

RELAX

Relax.

We are part of the universe and our lives are governed by the same laws that govern the whole of nature. And just like the rest of nature, we need to keep a balance. We need time to rest and recuperate, as do all other living things. Nature always takes her time. Everything of beauty and value took time to become that way. Think how long it takes for diamonds to be created for example, and the amount of time it takes a seed to grow to a majestic oak tree. In just the same way it takes time to build a healthy body and a positive outlook.

So don't be too hard on yourself. When we are relaxed and rested we are so much more productive than when we are tired or feeling under pressure. It makes a lot of sense. Have you noticed what happens when you are trying really hard to remember something? You don't remember it, do you? And then later when you've relaxed doing something else, what you were trying to remember will suddenly spring into your head without any effort. This is because our brain rhythms move into a slower mode (the alpha mode) when we are relaxed. Results come easily. That's the reason most of us have our best brain waves while engaged in activities where we are naturally relaxed.

During total relaxation all mental processes calm down and inner peace is achieved. When truly relaxed the mind is released from any agitation, doing or striving, and is focused in the present, so that we are troubled neither by memories from the past not plans for the future.

Physical relaxation is equally important for peak performance. When we relax our physical body, our whole metabolism comes into balance; our blood pressure drops, our breathing becomes deep and easy, and the organs in our body work harmoniously. We get the best results in our life when we find the elusive balance between effort and relaxation, between attachment and letting go. And we can take our lead from nature. The birds and the animals work, but they don't work day and night. They know when it's time to take a break. Nature knows a lot of things we only half know.

Our happiness is much more assured if we relax and let go of end results. Do you remember what happened when you tried so hard to impress the person you had a desperate crush on? I bet you tripped, or dropped your drink, or said something completely ridiculous from nerves. Probably the person you so admired ended up thinking you were a bit odd, meanwhile Sarah or David who you were yourself with and never tried to impress because you didn't fancy, thought you were wonderful. It seems if we only relax and let go of our desperation for something or someone, we are much more likely to be successful. It is the same with money. Most wealthy people are wealthy because they found something they love to do. Not because they woke up every morning with the sole objective of making money. When we find something we love to do, wealth tends to flow automatically.

In a sense we need to be able to live without something in order to have it. Once we relax and let go, we are in a position of greater power. Of course it is essential to put in hard work, but once we have put in our best effort, it is time to allow the results to happen in their own time. When you plant a seed you don't dig it up every day to see if it is growing. You know instinctively that you have done your bit, and that it's time to stand back, relax a while and let nature take its course. And then reap the rewards.

15

THINK HEALTHY

Think healthy!

What is a thought? Physicists tell us when we break down any object we get atoms and sub-atomic particles. These are pieces of matter vibrating at enormous speeds and are actually packets of energy. So the material world as we know it is really a mass of energies vibrating at different speeds.

Each time we have a thought our brain produces two things, energy and vibrations. Now science tells us that for every action there is an equal and opposite reaction. So for every thought we have, we produce a reaction or consequence. And considering that we may have around fifty thousand thoughts in one day, we are sending out a lot of vibrations and producing a lot of consequences. What we need to be aware of is that thoughts are real forces, they are energy.

Have you noticed that when you are feeling good about yourself, other people become very nice? That is because the world is a reflection of ourselves. When we hate ourselves, we hate everyone else. Our self image determines exactly how we will behave, who we will mix with, what we will try and what we will avoid. We live absolutely within the boundary of the picture we have of ourselves. If your self-image says that your co-ordination is excellent, you will pick up new sports easily. If your self-image says that you are hopeless at sports, then you will spend so much time worrying about dropping the ball, then that is exactly what you will do. And then you think 'There! That proves I am hopeless.'

A bad self-image says 'I don't deserve'. This results in a person subconsciously sabotaging his or her happiness. When exciting opportunities present themselves, perhaps a chance to take a holiday or learn a new skill, that person will consciously or subconsciously find reasons why it can't be done. So in order to achieve what we want and to be happy and healthy, each of us must work continually on maintaining a positive and healthy self-image.

Our subconscious is deeply intertwined with our self-concept. For example, when we are feeling badly about ourselves, we tend to take it out on ourselves through junk food binges, overindulgence in alcohol, illnesses and so on. Often this is not a conscious act, it is simply that our treatment of ourselves will automatically reflect how we feel about ourselves at any given moment. There is even evidence to suggest that people who have car accidents are often feeling badly towards themselves at that time, and that the accident may partly be a subconscious punishment.

Perhaps one of the most important principles about the mind is that you will always gravitate towards what you think about most. How often have you found yourself precisely in the situation you didn't want? You said to yourself 'Now if there is one thing I don't want to happen'...and then it did. When you think about something you move towards it. Even if you are thinking about something you don't, want you will move towards it. Have you ever said to yourself 'I mustn't forget that book' and then go and forget it? Your mind works in pictures, and so it sees a picture of you forgetting the book and it focuses on that result. When you tell yourself, 'I want to remember my book', you will have a mental picture of yourself remembering, and will in a much better position to remember. Your mind simply cannot work on the reverse of an idea. So when you say to your children, 'don't break aunties three thousand pound antique vase, you are asking for trouble! Always use language which paints pictures of the desired results in your mind.

Another dangerous tendency we have is to feel guilty. When we withhold forgiveness, we suffer. The 'guilty' person may not even be aware of what we are thinking. They are probably getting on with their life quite happily while there we are feeling upset, losing sleep, and setting ourselves up for an ulcer. The same goes for blaming other people for our problems. So long as we hold other people responsible for our unhappiness, we are effectively refusing to take action to solve our problems.

Forgiving ourselves is even more difficult. Many people spend their whole lives punishing themselves mentally and physically for what they perceive to be their own shortcomings. Some over-eat, some under-eat, some drink themselves into oblivion and so on. At the root of this suffering may be a belief system which says 'I have done a lot of bad things', 'I am guilty', or 'I don't deserve to be happy'. Well we do make mistakes, and sometimes do stupid things, yet we are still doing it the best way we know how. And while we are busy blaming ourselves we are avoiding the real issue which is to do something about the problem. Guilt achieves nothing, so throw it out! It is our choice whether we get on with our life, or whether we chain ourselves to grudges and upsets of the past.

Only you are in control of your own happiness since you decide what thoughts you think. To be happy, we need to concentrate on healthy, happy thoughts. Yet how often do we do the opposite? How often do we ignore a compliment and yet dwell on cruel remarks for weeks afterwards. Always remember, you are in control of your own mind. One person sees the pretty view and the other sees the dirty window. It is your choice what you see, and it is your choice what you think.

Being happy is a decision. Life will never be perfect, and happiness will not come up and tap you on the shoulder automatically when you win the lottery or get that car you always wanted. Life is about sometimes feeling exhilarated, sometimes feeling frustrated, sometimes achieving and sometimes missing out. The real key to contentment is in focusing our minds on the present. No matter what we did yesterday or what could happen tomorrow, now is really all we have. One of the beautiful things about young children is the way they become completely absorbed in the present moment. They are always totally involved in whatever they are devoting their energies to, whether it is building a sand castle, scribbling with crayons or watching a beetle. As we become adults we learn the dangerous art of thinking about and worrying about several things at the same time. We allow problems of the past and concerns about the future to crowd our present, and then we feel unhappy and under stress. And don't wait for happiness. A study showed that the average father spends about thirty seven seconds quality time per day with his child. No doubt many of these fathers have great plans for spending time with their loved ones 'when the house is finished', 'when the pressure is off at work'. But there are only 86,400 seconds available to us every day until we die. We have to decide if that is a limited time to make the most of what we've got, or whether we want to wish away the present, hoping for a better future.

Useful Addresses

Alexander Technique International

25 Marchels Drive
St Albans
AL1 4ZQ
01727 760 0767

Association of Chinese Acupuncture

1 Cline Road
London N11 2LX

0208 361 2121

Association of Medical Aromatherapists

Abergare
Rhu Point
HELENSBURGH
Strathclyde
G84 8NF
Tel: 0141 332 4924

Association of Natural Medicine

27 Braintree Road
Witham

Essex
CM8 2DD
Tel: 01376 502 762

Association of Reflexologists

5 Fore Street
Taunton
Somerset
TA1 1XX

01832 351010

British Acupuncture Association and Register

63 Jeddo Road
London
W12 9HQ

0208 735 0400

British Acupuncture Council

As above

British Chiropractic Association
59 Castle Street
READING
Berkshire

RG1 7SN
Tel: 0118 950 5950

British Herbal Medicine Association

BHMA
PO Box 583
Exeter
EX1 9GX

0845 680 1134

British Homeopathic Association

29 Park Street
Luton
LU1 3BE

0870 444 3950

British Medical Acupuncture Society

BMAS House
3 Winnington Court
Northwich
CW8 1AQ

01606 786 782

British Reflexology Association

Monks Orchard
WHITBOURNE
Worcestershire
WR6 5RB

01886 821207

Council for Complementary Medicine

10 Belgrave Square
LONDON
SW1 8PU

Council for Complimentary and Alternative Medicine

1 Harley Street
London W1G 9QD

Dr Edward Bach Centre

Mount Vernon
Bakers Lane
Brightwell Cum Sotwell
Oxfordshire
OX10 0PZ

Tel: 01491 834 678

European Chiropractors Union

C/O 9 Cross Deep Gardens
TWICKENHAM
Middlesex
TW1 4QZ
Tel: 0208 891 2546

Faculty of Homeopathy

Hahnemann House
29 Park Street West
Luton LU1 3BD

0870 444 3950

Foundation for Traditional Chinese Medicine

296 Tadcaster Road
York
YO24 1ET

01904 709688

GB Association of Homeopathic Vets
103 Golf Drive
Nuneaton
Warwickshire
CV11 6ND

GB Holistic Medical Association

0845 465 1056

Holistic Association of Reflexologists

5 Fore Street
Taunton
Somerset
TA1 1HX

01823 351010

Institute of Traditional Herbal Medicine & Aromatherapy

1 Laburnam lane
Burwell
Cambridgeshire
CB25 OEB

01638 741296

International Federation of Aromatherapists

61-63 Churchfield Road
Acton
London
W3 6AY
0208 992 9605

International Federation of Reflexologists

76-78 Edridge Road
CROYDON
Surrey
CR0 1EF
Tel: 0208 645 9134

International Institute of Reflexology

146 Upperthorpe
Walkely
Sheffield

01142 812100

National Institute of Medical Herbalists

Elm House
54 St Mar Ardens
EXETER
Devon
EX4 3BA
Tel: 01392 426 022

Reflexologists Society

39 Prestbury Road
Cheltenham

Gloucestershire
GL 52 2PT

01242 512 601

Scottish Chiropractic Association

Laigh Hatton Farm
Old Greenock Road
Bishopston
Renfrewshire
PA7 5PB

0141 404 0260

Scottish Institute of Reflexology

info@scottishreflexology.org

Society of Homeopaths

11 Brookfield
Duncan Close
Moulton Park
Northampton
NN3 6WL

0845 450 6611

The British Holistic Medical Association

PO Box 371
Bridgewater
Somerset
TA6 9BG
01278 722000

The Herb Society

PO Box 626
Banbury
OX16 6EY

01295 812 376

The Holistic Aromatherapy Foundation

contact@ihaf.co.uk

The Institute for Complementary Medicine

Unit 25 Tavern Key Business Centre
Sweden Gate
London SE16 7TX

0208 7231 5855

The National Consultative Council

39 Prestbury Road
CHELTENHAM
Gloucestershire
GL52 9PT
Tel: 01242 512 601

The Professional Association of Alexander Teachers

Room 706
The 'Big Pea'
120 Vyste street
Birmingham
B18 6NF

01746 761024

UK Homeopathic Medical Association

7 Darnley Road
Gravesend
Kent
DA11 ORY

560336

Emerald Publishing
www.emeraldpublishing.co.uk

106 Ladysmith Road
Brighton BN2 4EG

Other titles in the Emerald Series:

Law
Guide to Bankruptcy
Conducting Your Own Court case
Guide to Consumer law
Creating a Will
Guide to Family Law
Guide to Employment Law
Guide to European Union Law
Guide to Health and Safety Law
Guide to Criminal Law
Guide to Landlord and Tenant Law
Guide to the English Legal System
Guide to Housing Law
Guide to Marriage and Divorce
Guide to The Civil Partnerships Act
Guide to The Law of Contract
The Path to Justice
You and Your Legal Rights

Health
Guide to Combating Child Obesity

Asthma Begins at Home

Music
How to Survive and Succeed in the Music Industry

General
A Practical Guide to Obtaining probate
A Practical Guide to Residential Conveyancing
Writing The Perfect CV
Keeping Books and Accounts-A Small Business Guide
Business Start Up-A Guide for New Business
Finding Asperger Syndrome in the Family-A Book of
Answers

For details of the above titles published by Emerald go to:

www.emeraldpublishing.co.uk